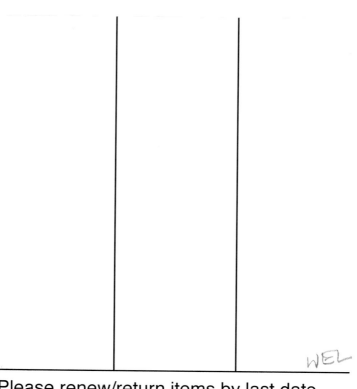

WEL

Please renew/return items by last date
shown. Please call the number below:

Renewals and enquiries: 0300 1234049

Textphone for hearing or
speech impaired users: 01992 555506

www.hertfordshire.gov.uk/libraries   Hertfordshire
L32

Moly Publishing

johnmolyneux.com

First published 2020 in the United Kingdom by Moly Publishing

ISBN 978-1-9161271-2-8 (print)
ISBN 978-1-9161271-3-5 (ebook)

A catalogue record for this book is available from the British Library

Printed in the United Kingdom

Cover design by Ken Leeder
Illustrations by Duncan Bullimore
Interior design and layout by Daisy Editorial

Disclaimer

Contents

About the author

John Molyneux has over 20 years' experience as a qualified and accredited sports therapist. He has developed a skill and passion for bringing exercise to those who struggle to maintain a regime or to exercise at all. He has particular expertise in working with age-related barriers, beginning with a gentle and appropriate introduction to exercise and gradually developing ability and confidence.

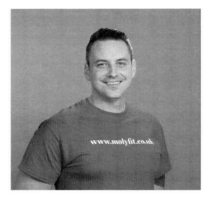

John firmly believes that exercise is accessible to anyone regardless of their age, ability or physical restrictions. This book is the product of his experience and is an easy-to-use guide for anyone who wants to acquire an exercise routine independently.

Before you start

If you've read my first book, *A Better You in Later Life*, welcome back! Are you engaging your core? I would like to think you are. If you're a new reader, you're welcome too, and you'll soon find out why your core is so important to being An Even Better You.

Whereas *A Better You in Later Life* was entry level to get you back into exercise, *An Even Better You* will step up the exercises and really get you to push the boundaries of what you think you are capable of achieving. Before, I took it easy on you, using exercises that would stretch and loosen off your body whilst keeping your spine neutral and your core engaged. Now, we are going to get your blood pumping and work your muscles to increase strength and total body fitness.

I want you to be aware that the exercises and routines in this book have a much greater difficulty level than the previous book. If you find an exercise too difficult or feel that it is having a negative effect, or is causing pain or discomfort, then stop. Please do not continue if you are in pain. Try to stretch or loosen off the area that is troubling you. If you are uncertain how to achieve this then visit my website https://www.molyfit.co.uk/ or seek help from a healthcare professional.

Test routine

To make sure that you will be able to tackle the contents of this book without causing any injury or setting off any pre-existing conditions, let's start with a little test routine: a warm-up then some exercises.

I have put all the routines and exercises covered in this book on my website, so if you are in any doubt on technique, please use the website for reference. The website is free to use. You will just need to enter your email address and choose a password to gain entry into My MolyFit to access the required exercises.

Warm-up

Let's start with the **Moly checklist**. You're going to be using this essential preparation a lot, so take some time to get it right.

Please look at the diagrams in the exercise reference at the end of this book to make sure you are doing the exercises properly.

- ▶ Feet hip distance apart
- ▶ Soft knees
- ▶ Activate core
- ▶ Neutral spine
- ▶ Open chest

Feet hip distance apart

Place your feet the same distance apart as your hips. This will position your feet directly under your hips. Now, make sure that your heels and toes are equal distance apart (feet parallel).

Soft knees

For this you will need to soften, not bend, your knees. You just need to relax your calf muscles slightly, so you feel the tension move out of the back of your legs and into your thighs. If done correctly, you will not feel any pressure in your knees, but just in the front of your thighs.

Activate core

Starting from your groin, gently pull your muscles in, up to your navel. Try not to make the action too strong; it should be just enough to feel your muscles activating, not straining. It is easy to overdo this exercise.

Neutral spine

Here, your lower back should feel comfortable. It should not be too arched, and it should not be too flat. It should be just right. If you are in the correct position then you shouldn't feel your lower back at all.

Open chest

Be mindful when opening your chest not to arch your lower back; it is easy to do. When you open your chest, you should feel your rib cage expanding and your shoulders gently travelling back. This will give you the feeling of your chest opening. You should feel your chest muscles opening from your sternum to your shoulders.

Exercises

March on the spot

With the Moly checklist in mind, start marching on the spot. I want you to do this for 5 minutes to get your blood flowing and warm up your body. Without a warm-up, it is easy to cause injury due to your muscles being tight. The purpose of a warm-up is to get blood into your muscles. Blood will give them oxygen for energy production and make sure that, when you begin the workout, they are loose and thus less prone to injury.

March on the spot with high knees and swing those arms for 5 minutes, taking in big deep breaths as you do.

Squat and reach

Start by standing up and using the Moly checklist. Activate your core and make sure your spine is neutral. Bend your elbows and place your hands in front of your chest, elbows behind your hands. Keep your eyes facing forward, fixed on something n front of you.

With your feet hip distance apart, toes very slightly facing out imagine you are sitting down on a chair and push your bottom as far back as you can. At the same time, push your hands forward until your arms are straight. As your bottom goes back, your knees will bend. Make sure your bottom goes no lower than your knees, and your knees no less than a 90-degree angle (thighs parallel to the floor). When you have reached the lowest point of the movement, hold the position for a few seconds, then gently stand back up, bringing your hands back to your chest and bending your elbows. Repeat this 10 times.

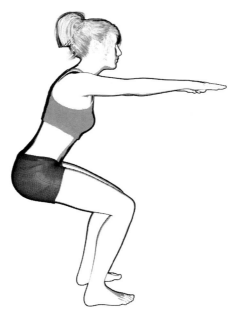

➲ Things to look out for:

Keep your eyes facing forward and don't look down. Also, be aware of what your knees are doing. It is absolutely normal for your body to try to cheat. This usually happens with your knees moving towards each other. It is a normal habit in which your mind is telling your body that you are better off doing so. Be aware of this and keep your knees equal distance apart throughout the entire exercise. Make sure that your knees do not travel forward past your toes. By keeping them just over your ankles, and pushing your bottom back, you will really engage your quads and gluteus muscles, keeping unwanted pressure out of your knees.

- ▶ Keep eyes facing forward.
- ▶ Knees stay behind toes.
- ▶ Push your bottom back.
- ▶ Maintain a neutral spine.
- ▶ You should feel this exercise mainly in your core, thighs and bottom.

Wall squat

This is an isometric exercise where the muscle and associated joint don't noticeably move or change. Isometric exercises are great if you have arthritis as they allow you to gain strength without upsetting your joints. This form of exercise can help you build up the strength required to progress onto other exercises.

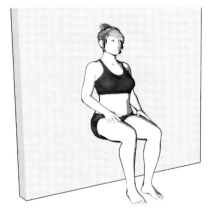

Make sure the wall you do this against is solid and can support your body weight. Place your back against a wall, making sure the surface is smooth with no protrusions. Gently walk your feet out to around 60cm (2 feet) from the wall (depending on your height). With your feet just wider than hip distance apart, slide your back down the wall, bending your legs until your thighs are at a 90-degree angle. Your bottom should not be lower than your knees. Make sure your knees are directly above your ankles, as the closer your feet are to the wall, the more pressure goes into your knees. With your arms straight down by your sides, try to hold this position for 30–60 seconds. Then, using your thighs, gently and slowly push yourself back up the wall into a standing position.

➲ Things to look out for:

► Keep your hips slightly higher than your knees.
► Make sure your knees are not further forward than your toes.
► Keep your feet at least hip distance apart.
► You should feel this in your thighs.

Straight arm plank

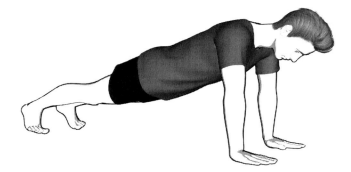

Again, this is an isometric strengthening. You need to be mindful of your core and keep a neutral spine. Start by getting down on the floor on all fours. With your fingers facing forward, place your hands directly under your shoulders. Make sure the insides of your elbows are facing each other. Reach your legs out behind you one at a time, onto bent toes. Tighten your buttocks and activate your core whilst maintaining a neutral spine. Keep your head and neck in line with your spine and hold the position for 30 seconds.

⮑ Things to look out for:

- ▶ Keep your hands directly under your shoulders.
- ▶ Keep your head in line with your bottom.
- ▶ You should not feel this in your back. If you do, activate your core or raise your bottom a little higher.

⮟ ⮟ ⮟

That is the end of the test routine. How did you get on? Was it too much or was it too easy? Did the exercises cause pain in any joints or muscles? This book is written to challenge your body. Together, we are really going to work on building your fitness levels. If you struggled to complete the exercises, think carefully whether continuing is yet right for you. We want to increase your strength and fitness, not set you back. You might need to do some preparatory work before you continue with this book. You can do that on my website using the 28-day courses in daily tasks.

Anyway, lecture over. Let's begin building An Even Better You.

Now let's stretch

We are going to complete an all-over body stretch just to make sure there are no problems lurking that you didn't know were there. This way, you can pick out the areas of your body that need attention so that, when you start the exercises, you are fully prepared and will not cause unnecessary injury.

During the stretches, I want you to listen to your body and feel what it is telling you. You should never feel pain when stretching. There is a big difference between a strong stretch and a painful stretch. Make sure there is no pain when you are stretching, either in your muscles or surrounding joints.

Here are some questions that I want you to ask yourself when you are doing each stretch:

- ► Can you perform the stretch whilst maintaining a neutral spine, and is your core activated?
- ► Using the illustrations provided, can your body position mirror the illustrations or is it cheating in some way? Remember, the body is lazy and will take shortcuts, trying to find the easiest way to do an exercise.
- ► Are you able to hold the stretch for 20 seconds and feel it in the desired location?
- ► Are you remembering to breathe? Holding your breath prevents oxygen from reaching your muscles. Without oxygen, your muscles stress and fatigue, which will restrict your stretches. Breathing will help relax your body, increase circulation and get rid of lactic acid (the waste from converting oxygen into energy in your muscles), making the stretch much more stretchy.

If you answer no to any of these questions during the stretch, try not to force it. Stay calm and patient, gently easing into your muscle whilst taking deep breaths. Keep persevering until you can answer yes to all before moving on.

Let's start with the door hinge, a great all-rounder that will quickly show you if there is any tension in your body.

The door hinge

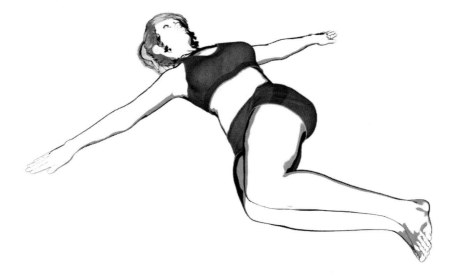

For this you will need a pillow. Lie on your side with your knees bent and your head on the pillow for support. With straight arms, palms together, place your arms out in front of you.

Now, with your legs pressed together and fixed on the floor, move your top arm all the way to the floor behind you. As you do so, let your eyes follow your fingertips. Do the action slowly and in a controlled way. If you rush, you can pull that tight muscle that had been hiding unaware. As soon as the back of your hand hits the floor (whether it is able to depends on your flexibility), take a breath and try to open your chest, stretching your muscles by lowering the active shoulder to the floor. When ready, bring your arm back. Repeat this 10 times on each side. If you are struggling to reach the floor, don't push too hard. Just try to go a little further each time. Unless there is a real problem, you should be able to reach the floor by the tenth time.

You will feel the stretch of this exercise in the area that is tight. The usual suspects are chest, arms, hips, ribs or lower back. Make a note of where you feel the tension pulling and work on stretching those muscles.

➲ Things to look out for:

► Keep your knees together with your bottom leg staying on the floor.
► Don't rush, and breathe as you do this exercise. This will help open your rib cage and relieve any tension in your ribs.
► Make sure your eyes follow your fingertips to stretch your neck muscles.
► Keep your arms straight. This will maximise the stretch in your muscles and tendons.

Glute stretch

Lie on your back with your right ankle on your left knee. Keep your shoulders down, relax and breathe. Using both arms, place your hands behind your left leg, just under your bent knee and gently pull your leg towards your chest. Try to keep the angle of

11

your left knee around 90 degrees. You are aiming for your left knee to be above your navel. The stretch should feel strong and obvious in the centre of your right buttock. You should only feel it in the glute. If you can feel it anywhere else, stop. It may be that tight muscles elsewhere are inhibiting the stretch and need to be stretched themselves before you can progress. Don't force it. Hold the stretch for 20 seconds, then repeat with the other leg.

You may not be physically able to take hold of your knee with both hands because of complications elsewhere in your body. If this is the case, place a towel around your leg and pull on the towel to bring your leg towards your chest.

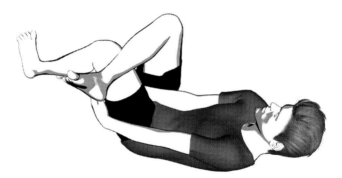

➲ Things to look out for:

► Ease into the stretch, don't force it.
► Try to keep you head down on the floor.
► Keep the leg you are pulling into your body with a 90-degree bend at your knee.

Gluteus medius stretch

Avoid this exercise if you have had a hip replacement.

This is the best stretch to target the gluteus medius as it doesn't put pressure on your spine. If your body allows it, you will feel the stretch radiating from your bottom into your lower back. However, for this stretch to be beneficial, everything else has to be working correctly. Quite often, the muscles in your legs, back and bottom are too tight so inhibit this stretch. Wear and tear in your hips also restrict this stretch. If that's the case, you will feel it in your groin, not where you are meant to. Give it a go, but if you can feel it anywhere other than where you are meant to, stop.

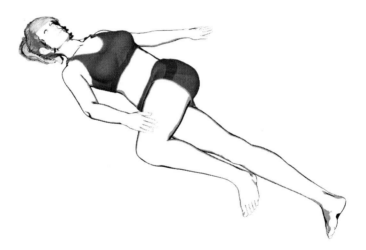

Lie on your back with your right leg flat. Bring your left leg across your right leg and place your left foot so that it is on the outside of your right knee. Make sure the sole of your left foot is not on the floor. You want the inside of your foot and ankle facing the floor.

Anchor your body into your left shoulder and place your right hand on your left knee. Gently pull your left knee to the floor. Don't pull too hard or you will turn your pelvis. As soon as you feel a stretch, stop and hold for 20 seconds. Your knee should never touch the floor. It doesn't have to move much to get the stretch. If you try too hard there is a good chance of setting off another muscle somewhere else causing an unwanted spasm. Less is more with this one! Repeat with the other leg.

➲ Things to look out for:

▸ Anchor your body with your shoulders.
▸ Your knee should not touch the floor, so don't force it to.

Hamstring stretch

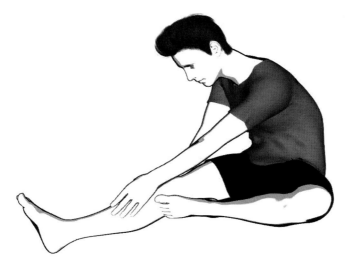

Sit on the floor with your legs out wide. Roll up a towel and place it under your right knee. Place your left foot on the inside of your right knee and, if you can, let your left knee fall down to the floor. Slide both hands down your right leg towards your foot. You should feel this stretch at the back of your thigh, between your knee and bottom. When you feel a strong stretch, hold for 20 seconds. Repeat on the other side.

➲ Things to look out for:

▸ Your active leg (the one you are stretching) should remain soft at the knee, otherwise your calf will take over and you will feel the stretch there instead.
▸ If you can't reach your toes then slide your hands as far down your leg as they will naturally go, hold that position for 20 seconds, then try to slide a little further down towards your foot.
▸ Alternatively, for a really strong stretch, place a towel around the heel of your active foot and use it to pull yourself towards your foot.

Hip flexor stretch

Kneel with your right knee on the floor and your left leg at a 90-degree angle in front of you. Put your right hand on your right hip and your left hand on your left knee. Maintain a neutral spine, keeping your back straight. Keeping your right knee on the floor, lean forward, squeezing your glutes whilst shifting your body weight forward.

You will feel the stretch on the active side, in this case the right. The stretch will work the muscles from the top of your thigh down towards your knee. Hold for 20 seconds, then repeat on the other side.

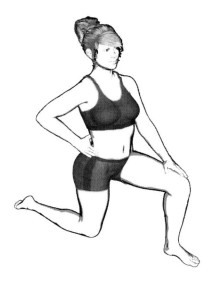

➲ Things to look out for:

► As you shift your body forward, maintain a straight back with neutral spine.

Cat stretch

Gently get down onto the floor, onto your hands and knees. With your arms and legs parallel, the same distance apart, arch your spine to the ceiling, pushing your belly up and in. Gently lower your head to stretch your neck. Feel the stretch in the muscles that run from your neck to the base of your spine. Hold this stretch for 20 seconds, and remember to breathe.

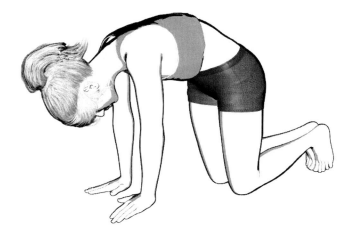

➲ Things to look out for:

► The main area where you should feel this is your back. As you arch up you should feel the muscles stretching on both sides of your spine.
► Keep your head down so the stretch also works in your neck.

Downward dog-ish

This is an adaptation of one of the most recognised yoga stretches, the downward dog. It strengthens your arms and thighs whilst stretching your calves, spine, hips and hamstrings. Another great exercise to show you where your weaknesses are. I am using this mainly as a calf stretch so won't go into the full technicalities of the position and alignment. Sorry if this offends any yoga fans!

On your hands and knees, place your knees directly under your hips with your hands shoulder width apart, wrists slightly in front of your shoulders, fingers forward. Activate your core and, with a neutral spine, breathe in. As you exhale, tuck in your toes and lift your knees off the floor. Reach your bottom towards the ceiling and try to straighten your legs. Gently push your heels down towards the floor, feeling the stretch in your calves. Hold for 20 seconds and then gently lower yourself back onto all fours.

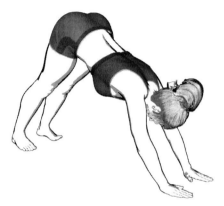

◯ Things to look out for:

▶ This exercise puts a lot of pressure on your hands and shoulders, so avoid it if you have carpal tunnel or a bad back. Make sure your spine stays neutral.
▶ Don't rush to get up after this as you may feel dizzy with the rush of blood going to your head.
▶ Done properly this is an excellent exercise, but it is hard to execute correctly. It is definitely worth going to a yoga class to see how it is done if you enjoy this stretch and want to learn more.

Quad stretch

Don't do this exercise if you have had a knee replacement.

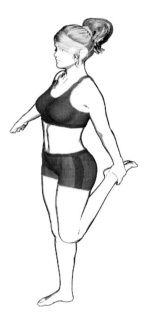

Firstly, you will need to support yourself on something appropriate that can fully take your body weight. Standing tall and using the Molyfit checklist, use one hand to bend your leg back at the knee by holding your ankle and taking your foot towards your bottom. The other hand should be holding something suitable for support. Standing tall, when your foot has gone back as far as possible, push your pelvis forward keeping your knees together. Try not to let the bent knee travel forwards. Hold the stretch for 20 seconds, then repeat on the other side.

➲ Things to look out for:

▶ If you struggle to grab your ankle, extend your reach by using a towel around your ankle to pull your leg back.
▶ This stretch should only be felt in your thigh, never your knee.

Hug the tree stretch

Stand up with your feet hip distance apart, soften your knees and keep a neutral spine. Imagine that there is a massive tree in front of you with a large trunk and give it a cuddle. Hug it with your fingers clasped together and elbows bent.

Feel your trapezius muscles in your upper back pulling away from each other and pulling outwards away from your spine. Draw that feeling into your shoulders and down your arms. Gently lower your head so you are looking at the floor, as this will stretch the trapezius further. When you are happy that you can feel an effective stretch, hold it for 20 seconds.

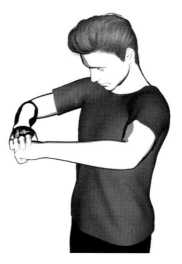

➲ Things to look out for:

► The tree wants to be a big one! Think oak not acer!

Chest stretch

Stand tall with a neutral spine, feet hip distance apart. Open your chest and relax your shoulders. Activate your core. Make a fist behind you in the small of your back and gently try to bring your elbows and shoulder blades together. Hold for 20 seconds, taking in big breaths as you do.

Breathe in through your nose and out through your mouth. Keep your eyes forward, trying not to bend your neck. You will feel your chest muscles stretching from your sternum towards your shoulders. You may also feel something in your shoulders as they stretch, but be careful and look out for pain. If your shoulders are too tight or carrying an injury, the stretch will aggravate.

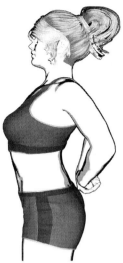

➲ Things to look out for:

▸ Keep your eyes facing forward and activate your core so that you don't arch your back.
▸ This is an exercise where you can easily hyperextend your back if your core isn't switched on!

Hands to ceiling

When was the last time you stretched your hands to the ceiling? It fascinates me how many people can't fully extend their arms in an upward direction. The action just seems to get lost as we age! With this in mind, let's give it a go.

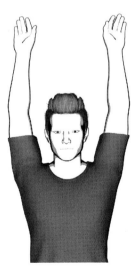

Use the Moly checklist and, without arching your back, reach your hands to the ceiling. Starting from your shoulders, push through into your elbows, then your wrists and all the way into your fingertips.

21

Are your arms straight? Can you push through your fingers and fully extend them? If you can't then this is one to practise. Feel where the resistance in your body is coming from and stretch that area independently.

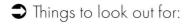 Things to look out for:

▶ If you are struggling with this exercise, don't force it. It is easy to try too hard and end up pulling something.
▶ Make sure you maintain a neutral spine and don't arch your lower back.
▶ Keep your eyes forward and avoid looking up, as this can cause imbalance and dizziness.

⊿ ⊿ ⊿

Understanding your body during exercise

Working to heart rate (HR)

It is important to understand what's happening to your body when you exercise and to be able to measure your effort levels. As you exercise, the blood in your body moves towards the muscles that you are using. This is why it is said don't train just after a meal. When you eat, blood goes into your stomach to aid digestion. If you exercise just after a meal, the blood leaves your stomach and redirects to your muscles, leaving the job half done, which gives you indigestion.

Muscles need oxygen to produce the energy required for exercise. The harder you work out, the more oxygen your muscles need. Your heart beats more quickly to transport the blood, and your breathing rate increases. The heart is a muscle. As you get fitter, your heart gets stronger. If you train too hard, you will put a strain on your heart as it can't cope with the demand. Likewise, if you train too little, you will not challenge your body and your fitness will not improve.

It is all about balance: knowing your body's strengths and also its limitations. Recognising when to stop is just as important as knowing when to push. Listen to your body. When your heart starts beating rapidly and you can feel your chest tightening as your breathing increases, you are training too hard. If you feel like you could do the exercise all day and your breathing hasn't changed much, then step it up until it does.

This is where working to heart rate comes into play. It's the perfect way to understand your effort levels in a safe and accurate way. There are plenty of devices now that will monitor your heart rate, unlike the old-fashioned way where you had to stop training, measure your pulse for 30 seconds and multiply the reading by two. Now all you have to do is glance at your wrist. When you work to heart rate you never want to exceed your maximum heart rate (MHR). Working any higher will put unnecessary stress on your heart.

Your MHR is calculated by deducting your age from 220. So, if you are 70 years old, your MHR is 150 beats per minute (bpm). When exercising, your target heart rate zone is 50–85% of MHR. A 70-year-old person should therefore have a heart rate of 75–128 beats per minute when exercising.

One thing to mention that often gets overlooked is medication and heart rate. Some medications have side effects that will lower your resting heart rate. An example of this is blood pressure pills. You may find your resting heart rate is 60 bpm or lower. If this is the case, talk to a health professional. You may have to recalculate the heart rate figures for these circumstances. If you are targeting a working heart rate of 120 bpm but your natural heart rate has been lowered by medication, you can easily blow a gasket trying to get there, so you will need to reduce the figures to accommodate this change.

Rate of perceived exertion (RPE)

The rate of perceived exertion is a way of measuring exercise intensity that gives you awareness of effort. Usually, trainers will ask you to imagine a scale between zero and 10, zero being no effort and 10 being very, very hard. They will then ask where your effort level is on that scale. It is a way of looking at our effort levels without the need for a heart rate monitor. I have modified the scale to show what I expect of you whilst exercising. Try to keep your effort in between 4 and 7 on the scale, which is the equivalent of working to 50–85% of MHR.

1. Not even trying
2. I'm trying a little, but if I'm honest, not much
3. There might be some effort involved
4. Well, I'm getting warmer
5. Something's happening
6. I can feel my muscles and my body is letting me know
7. I'm starting to sweat but am still talking and breathing
8. 'Ave it! I can really feel this now
9. Breathing is getting difficult, and I'm not sure how long I will last
10. Crikey, I hope my affairs are in order

If you haven't got a device to measure your heart rate and you can't be bothered with the faff of counting your pulse, then the RPE is the next best thing to monitor your effort levels.

What is the difference between fitness and health?

This book is not the place to get into a detailed discussion on the differences between fitness and health, and I'm lacking the PhD to do it any justice! I do, however, think it is important to tap into it slightly, as without a basic understanding, how can you strive to achieve either? Here are my basic descriptions:

Fitness means improving cardiovascular function and muscle gain; the condition of being physically fit and healthy.

Health is a state of complete physical, mental and social wellbeing and not merely the absence of disease.

Health is therefore not just an absence of disease, but also a state of wellness. When you look at total fitness and health, you see the two aspects cannot exist without the other. Total fitness means being fit and well in mind, body and spirit. What is the point of having a fit body and not using your brain? I once met a doctor who told me that the key to maintaining an active old age is to take up dancing and learn a language. This is because our brain needs as much exercise as our body. As we get older, we need to be mindful of exercise for the benefits, such as more energy, more oxygen circulation for the body, and better health and immune system. Total fitness is a lifestyle. It is about taking control of life and living it.

Total fitness

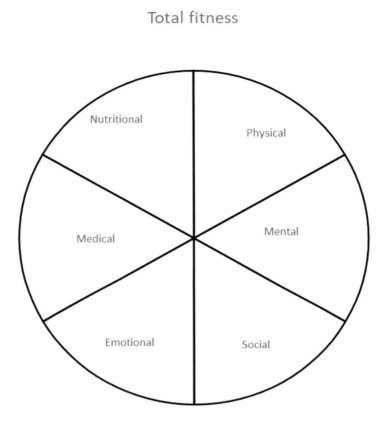

To achieve total fitness, you need to look further than how long you can hold a wall squat and how many biscuits you had with your tea. You need to factor in your emotional state, relationships and communities. For instance, taking part in a group activity is a great motivational tool. It will enhance your performance through competition, increase your commitment and really get those endorphins going. Yes, working out alone increases endorphins, but working out in a group increases them even more. A group setting can lead to the release of endorphins before exercise has begun. Smiling has even been shown to increase endorphin levels! Think of endorphins as the positivity hormone. They are natural chemicals produced by the body to relieve stress and pain. Through regular exercise, endorphins will help to reduce stress, anxiety and depression, improve sleep and boost self-esteem, all vital for achieving total fitness.

⋏ ⋏ ⋏

Let's get back to the purpose of this book: improving your fitness and improving cardiovascular function and muscle strength.

Fitness can be broken down into separate components.

Components of fitness

Aerobic fitness: Your body's ability to take in oxygen and use it to produce energy for your muscles. This uses your heart and lungs, your circulatory system.

Muscular strength: Maximum force of a muscle or group of muscles in a single contraction.

Flexibility: Fluid and full range of movement of a joint.

Muscular endurance: Ability of muscles to work against resistance for an extended period.

Body composition: Ratio of fat to muscle.

Nutrition: Balanced diet with optimum nutrient levels.

Relaxation: Reduction or elimination of unnecessary tension.

Neuromuscular efficiency: Motor, mental and muscular integration.

Posture: Balance between strength and flexibility.

Skill-related components

Speed: Calculated by distance divided by time, speed is the maximum rate at which you are able to perform a movement. To increase speed, you need power and strength.

Power: The ability to move weight with speed, to exert maximum force as quickly as possible.

Agility: The ability to quickly change body position or direction. Agility requires the combination of balance, speed, strength and coordination.

Reaction time: The ability to respond quickly to a stimulus. The ageing process slows down reaction time, so it is important to work at it.

Balance: The ability to stay in control of body movement, statically when still or dynamically when moving.

Coordination: The integration of eye, hand and foot movements. Moving your body parts under control.

All of the components of fitness will naturally decrease with age. Regular exercise will compensate for this, reducing the risk of disease and falls. All the research shows that it's never too late to begin and to gain the health benefits from a more active lifestyle. We will make a start on working on all the components of fitness in a while. Before then, let's talk about the common diseases affecting the over 65s we are trying to prevent by building An Even Better You.

Illnesses affecting the over 65s and how exercise can help

Too much of my thinking time goes into cancer. The one negative and hideous side of working with older adults is that I have lost so many people that I care about because of it. Half of us will get it, and I want to know that, when we do, treatment will be available there and then, with no delays. So many diseases affecting the over 65s are preventable if you are engaged in a regular exercise regime. It would take such a burden off the NHS if we all did our bit and moved a bit more. Exercise can reduce your risk of major illness such as heart disease, stroke, type 2 diabetes and some cancers by up to 50%. Exercise can lower your risk of early death by up to 30%. Come on, sit less and move more! Here are the illnesses that I want to beat the drum about.

Heart disease: Regular exercise can help improve your heart health. Exercise can lower your blood pressure, thereby lowering your risk of dying of heart disease, and lower the risk of it progressing.

Diabetes: Diabetes now costs the NHS over £1 billion a year. About 90% of diabetes is type 2, which can usually be reversed through cutting back on sugar and exercising regularly. Just reducing sugar in tea can help. People in the UK drink on average 28 cups of tea a week. Do you take sugar in your tea? Do the maths.

Asthma: Exercise can help control the frequency and severity of asthma attacks.

Back pain: Strengthening your core and looking after your posture will stop unnecessary pressure going into your back. Exercise will increase your strength and endurance by improving muscle function.

Arthritis: Exercise can help reduce pain, and it will help the joints by maintaining muscle strength around the affected areas. It can reduce joint stiffness and improve physical function.

Dementia: People who exercise regularly reduce the risk of developing heart disease and stroke, high blood pressure, type 2 diabetes and obesity, all of which are associated with developing dementia.

The best thing about exercise is that it is free. By helping ourselves, we can help others by reducing the burden on the NHS from illnesses that can be preventable. The leading causes of death among the over 75s in England are:

- ▶ cancer
- ▶ chronic heart disease
- ▶ stroke
- ▶ dementia
- ▶ chronic obstructive pulmonary disease (COPD).

Let's work down the list.

Cancer

Cancer is a condition where cells in a specific part of the body grow and reproduce uncontrollably. The cancer cells can invade and destroy the surrounding healthy tissue. In the UK, the most common types are breast, lung, prostate and bowel cancer. We know half of us (1 in 2) will get cancer. Exercise will not stop you getting cancer, or will it? It is well documented that exercise can contribute to the prevention of bladder, breast, colon, oesophagus, kidney, stomach and uterine cancer. Exercise can help improve survival rates for certain cancers. The recommended amount of exercise for older adults is 150 minutes of moderate activity a week (such as walking, gardening, swimming) or 75 minutes of vigorous activity a week (running, sport, climbing stairs).

Chronic heart disease

Chronic heart disease is a condition in which the heart has trouble pumping blood around the body. It is caused by:

▶ **coronary artery disease** (a build-up of fatty deposits in the arteries that reduce blood flow and cause a heart attack)
▶ **a heart attack** (a blockage that stops the heart getting the oxygen it needs from blood; without oxygen, the heart tissue dies, causing permanent damage)
▶ **high blood pressur**e (the pressure of blood on the arteries; if it's high, there is a strain on the heart as it works harder).

Chronic heart disease can be down to your genes, but it is also brought on by bad diet, lack of exercise, being overweight and smoking. Regular exercise lowers the risk by 35%.

Stroke

There are two main causes of a stroke. The first is when the blood supply to the brain is cut off. As with a heart attack, the brain cells die without oxygen. The other cause is where a weakened blood vessel supplying the brain bursts. High blood pressure, high cholesterol and diabetes increase the risk of having a stroke, so by exercising, losing weight and watching your diet, you can greatly reduce the risk.

Dementia

Dementia is not a natural part of ageing! Dementia is a group of related symptoms, a syndrome. Dementia is a decline of brain function that can cause problems with carrying out daily activities, memory loss, mental sharpness, mood and judgement, to name just a few. Alzheimer's disease is the most common type, affecting 62% of people diagnosed. Taking regular exercise can reduce the risk of developing Alzheimer's disease by 45%.

COPD

COPD is a group of lung conditions that cause difficulty breathing. The main cause is smoking but you can get it without being a smoker. Exercise will not cure it, but inactivity will cause a decline. Exercise can improve physical endurance and strengthen the respiratory muscles, which will lead to a greater tolerance when you exert yourself.

⋏ ⋏ ⋏

As you can see, with the leading causes of death among the over 75s there is a common theme. If you exercise, you greatly reduce your risk of getting them. The sad fact is that, as a nation – not just those over the age of 65 – we could all do better.

Benefits of a daily walk

Walking can help combat all of the diseases and illnesses I have covered so far, and it's free!

You don't have to pound the pavements for hours. Just 10 minutes a day is better than no minutes a day. As mentioned earlier, the exercise guidelines for people over 65 are to do at least 150 minutes of moderate-intensity activity a week, or 75 minutes of vigorous-intensity activity if you are already active, or a combination of both. So, 10 minutes walking every day equates to 70 minutes of your weekly quota.

The average walking speed is three miles an hour. Depending on your fitness level, this may or may not be fast enough to gain the best benefit. If you want to know what speed is right for you, either use the RPE scale and walk to about a level 5 or 6, or use a heart rate monitor and get your heart rate up to around 60% of MHR.

Walking daily has many benefits:

► strengthens your heart
► burns calories
► lowers blood sugar levels
► eases joint pain
► increases circulation (and so boosts energy)

▶ boosts your immune system
▶ improves your mood by reducing anxiety and negativity
▶ strengthens and tones your muscles
▶ airs out your soul and clears your head (so the little grey cells can work properly).

So, what are you waiting for? Activate your core, heel to toe, and walk, walk, walk.

So, what's all this 10,000 steps a day business all about?

According to legend, the 10,000 steps a day came about because of a marketing campaign in Japan for the 1964 Tokyo Olympics. In the run-up to the games, a company came up with a step-counting device, which they marketed to the health conscious. Based on the work of Dr Yoshiro Hatano, it was an early pedometer and counted 10,000 steps. Dr Hatano was worried that the Japanese people were not active enough and thought if he could convince them to increase their daily steps from 4,000 to 10,000 then they would burn an extra 500 calories a day, keeping them slim.

We all have different stride lengths but, on average, walking 10,000 steps a day is around five miles. You can argue for and against the 10,000-step method. There are so many less time-consuming and efficient ways of getting fit, but at the end of the day, it's down to personal choice.

If this method works for you then great, do it. Better to do something you enjoy than be forced into an activity you don't (so won't do). You have to enjoy your fitness activity. That way, you will be more inclined to get off your derrière and do it.

Why strength and flexibility are so important in later life

In the UK, falls are the most common cause of injury-related deaths in people over the age of 75. This is why it is so important to keep an eye on the components of fitness, to try to reduce this horrible statistic. Falls occur because of balance problems and muscular weakness. Poor vision and long-term health conditions such as heart disease, dementia and low blood pressure also cause falls. Obviously, exercise will not help your vision, but it certainly will help the other conditions. Low blood pressure is a condition that is often overlooked, as high blood pressure often steals the limelight. Low blood pressure causes dizziness and light-headedness, blurred vision, confusion and fainting, so it can be instrumental in causing falls.

Throughout the day, blood pressure varies. It can go up or down depending on body position, breathing rhythm, stress levels, medications you take, exercise, caffeine intake and other food and drinks. Blood pressure is usually lowest at night and rises sharply in the morning. We are all different and, in some people, low blood pressure is normal and causes no symptoms, but a sudden fall in blood pressure can be dangerous. It causes dizziness and fainting when the brain doesn't get enough oxygen due to lack of blood supply. The causes of low blood pressure vary but a common one is dehydration, so make sure you have at least 1.2 litres (six glasses) of water a day, especially when exercising. Low blood pressure is more common in older adults who take certain medications. Those that cause low blood pressure are diuretics (water pills), beta blockers, antidepressants, and drugs for Parkinson's disease, enlarged prostate and erectile dysfunction.

To avoid falls, the two things to look out for if you have low blood pressure are standing up from a seated position and going to the toilet in the night. Both of these can cause postural hypotension. This is a sudden drop in blood pressure when you stand from a seated or lying position, and it's worse at night because your blood pressure naturally lowers as you sleep. The trick is to be mindful of this and don't rush. Stand up slowly and wait a few seconds for the blood to flow around your body and into your brain. You can even try marching on the spot for a few seconds to help.

Muscle weakness as we age

Unfortunately, atrophy is a natural process of growing old. The older you get, the faster your muscles waste away, especially with underuse. From birth until your 30s, muscles grow stronger. After that, you start to lose muscle mass and function. From the age of 40, you can lose muscle mass at a rate of 5% a decade. Even if you stay active it will still happen, so if you are not active, it happens more. If you exercise and keep your muscles as strong as possible, this will help. It will help reduce frailty and the possibility of falls and other damage.

The best form of exercise for this is strength training and, as I said in the first book, the best piece of equipment for that is *you*. Strength training will help you maintain your balance, mobility and energy levels.

To keep your muscles strong, you have to fuel them. Muscles will not grow without protein. Protein is used by the body for growth and repair. For example, if you lift weights to gain strength and don't increase your protein, you won't achieve much muscle gain, and the same applies if you take protein without lifting weights. The two go hand in hand. To increase strength and muscle mass, you need strength training and to increase your protein intake, and you can do this with protein-rich foods or supplements.

It is always advisable to seek advice when changing your diet. In a healthy body, increasing protein is fine, but if your liver and kidneys are a bit past their best, excess protein can add to the damage. Having too much protein can cause waste to build up in your blood, which will put excess stress on your liver and kidneys. If you do have a liver or kidney problem, the amount of protein you need will be affected by this, as well as by your body size and the amount of protein in your urine. Like everything, it's better to check with a health professional first.

To combat atrophy and falls, I have included plenty of strength-building exercises that we will cover in the 8-week exercise plan, the next chapter in the book. We will also really work on your flexibility. Flexibility is key to remaining active and independent. Muscles shorten with age and, in doing so, will decrease the range of motion in your joints. Going back to the hands to the ceiling stretch (seeing if you can fully stretch your arms to the ceiling without arching your back), this is not an action you naturally do on a daily basis, so there is bound to be some muscle in your body that is pulling or niggling. If you have one tight muscle then you will have others. Tight muscles cause habits that lead to other complications such as joint pain and even reduced circulation. A few stretches a day will solve this, but you need to know where to stretch first. You do this by listening to your body and feeling where the tension is coming from. Niggles are your body's way of letting you know something needs to be done. If left, a minor issue that could have been easily fixed can become a major issue that takes months to recover from, so best to nip it in the bud.

By improving your flexibility you will:

▸ improve your physical performance
▸ make daily tasks easier
▸ have fewer injuries as your muscles can withstand more stress
▸ take the stress out of your joints so you will be in less pain
▸ improve your posture and balance.

Now let's roll out the mat and begin the 8-week course.

The 8-week course

Mountain climbers to the rescue

This 8-week course is designed to be done every day and will prepare you to tackle mountain climbers. I love this exercise as it covers everything in one and only takes 20 seconds! Mountain climbers will increase your strength, cardiovascular fitness and all of the other components of fitness other than nutrition.

The 8-week course will go a long way to helping you reduce your risk of type 2 diabetes, cardiovascular disease and dementia by increasing your fitness. We will really work on your strength, flexibility and posture.

Your starting point

Before we begin, use the tools on the next pages to take some measurements so you can compare the results when you have finished the 8-week course.

Waist-to-hip ratio

The waist-to-hip ratio (WHR) is an easy way of measuring fat distribution, indicating overall health. It is the circumference of your waist, divided by the circumference of your hips. If you carry more weight around your middle than your hips, you are classed as an apple shape and may have a higher risk of developing health conditions such as type 2 diabetes and cardiovascular disease.

First you will need to measure your waist. Stand straight and breathe out, then measure your waist just above the belly button, where it is smallest.

To measure your hips, place the tape measure around the widest part of your hips, usually across your buttocks.

To calculate your WHR, divide your waist measurement by your hip measurement.

Enter your results in the table below.

Date	Waist cm	Hip cm	WHR cm (w/h)
Example	*94*	*102*	*0.92*
Before 8-week course			
After 8-week course			

Having a WHR of over 1.0 may increase the risk of conditions that relate to being overweight.

A healthy WHR is thought to be:

► 0.85 or less for women
► 0.9 or less for men.

Resting heart rate (RHR)

To take your RHR either use your device or count your pulse. First you need to rest for at least 5 minutes, so sit down, relax and breathe. If you are counting your pulse, the easiest place to find it is in your neck.

► Press your first and second finger to the side of your neck, just under your jaw, beside your windpipe.
► Press your skin lightly to feel your pulse. Move your fingers around if you can't find it.

Count the number of beats for 30 seconds and multiply by two to give you the number of times your heart beats per minute.

Date	RHR
Before 8-week course	
After 8-week course	

Blood pressure

To measure your blood pressure you will need a special device. The average cost is around £10–20 but it is a good investment. You may have no symptoms of high blood pressure until it has majorly damaged your heart and arteries, which is why it's called the silent killer.

To take your blood pressure, sit down with your back supported and with uncrossed legs. Try not to hold your breath as this will give you a higher reading. Place the cuff around your upper arm, against your skin, with the arrow on the artery (just inside the head of your bicep towards your body). Try to relax and don't talk as this can also increase the reading.

Blood pressure is measured in mmHg. There are two readings, top and bottom. The top (systolic) is the pressure when your heart pushes out. The bottom (diastolic) is the pressure when your heat rests between beats. Normal blood pressure is between 90/60mmHg and 120/80mmHg. High blood pressure is 140/90mmHg or higher. Low blood pressure is 90/60mmHg or lower. If your reading is in the high or low figures, definitely talk to your doctor, exercise or not.

Date	Blood pressure reading
Before 8-week course	
After 8-week course	

Recovery heart rate

Target heart rate (beats per minute) zones during exercise are:

Age range	Target heart rate bpm (60–80% MHR)
50–59	102–136
60–69	96–128
70–79	90–120
80–89	84–112
90–99	78–104
100+	72–96

Finally, measure how your heart reacts to exercise. You have already taken your resting heart rate, now let's see how much it increases during a fitness test. All I want you to do is march on the spot for 5 minutes. Use the range table and try to get your heart rate into the target zone for your age bracket. Marching on the spot might not be enough, so you might have to go for a brisk walk or tackle some stairs. Please do not blow a gasket trying to get your heart rate there. Be sensible and listen to your body. If the target heart rate is too much for you, recognise this and stop. You can still measure your recovery time without hitting the zones!

When you have finished the 5 minutes of exercise, take your post-exercise heart rate straight away, using the methods discussed earlier. Sit down and recover for 2 minutes after completing the exercise and then take your recovery heart rate.

Date	Resting heart rate	Heart rate after 5 mins marching (post-exercise HR)
Before 8-week course		
After 8-week course		

Your recovery heart rate is the speed at which you heart rate returns to normal after exercise. It is a measure of fitness because people who are fit recover more quickly. However, if you are on medications that affect heart rate then don't use RHR as a fitness measurement as it is unfair for the reasons discussed earlier.

To calculate your recovery heart rate, subtract your two-minute recovery heart rate from the heart rate you took immediately after exercising. The faster your heart rate recovers, the healthier and fitter your heart is.

Date	Heart rate after 2 mins recovery	Recovery heart rate (rate after exercise minus rate after 2 mins recovery)
Before 8-week course		
After 8-week course		

If the difference between the two numbers is:

- less than 22, your biological age is older than your calendar age
- 22–52, your biological and calendar age are the same
- 53–65, your biological age is slightly younger than your calendar age
- 59–65, your biological age is moderately younger than your calendar age
- 66 or more, well done, you're looking fabulous darling! Your biological age is a lot younger than your calendar age.

The first minute of recovery is the most important. Your heart rate should drop by at least 12 beats after exercise. Any less than that is abnormal and indicates a lack of fitness or maybe cardiovascular disease. It's definitely worth talking to your GP if this is the case.

Let's get started

Right, it's now time to blow away the cobwebs and get your blood pumping. This exercise plan is designed to be done daily. However, you may be using muscles that haven't seen any action in a while, so don't be surprised if you get some aches. Listen to your body and know when to stop if you feel unwell or are pushing yourself too hard. Remember to breathe, maintain a neutral spine and drink water. If there is a particular exercise that is bothering you, use the advice on my website to ease your muscles off (https://www.molyfit.co.uk/), and if that doesn't work, leave out that particular exercise. There is a lot of floor work involved so you might also want to invest in a mat.

General strength

March on the spot: 5 minutes

March on the spot or go for a gentle walk to warm up for 5 minutes. Remember the Moly checklist: keep your core activated with a neutral spine. Keep your chest open with big, deep breaths. If you are walking, remember heel to toe.

Tea towel behind the neck: 30 seconds

Sit in a correct chair (bottom not lower than your knees) with your spine away from the back of the chair. Have your feet hip distance apart and your knees bent at a 90-degree angle. This is important because, if your feet are pulled back behind your knees, it engages the back of the thighs, which will pull on your back. Now hold the tea towel by each end above your head. Keep it taut but don't pull too hard. Engage your core and make sure your spine is neutral. Keep your eyes facing forward and pull the tea towel down to the base of your neck, keeping it straight without a bend. Then pull it back up again to the starting position. Repeat the exercise for 30 seconds.

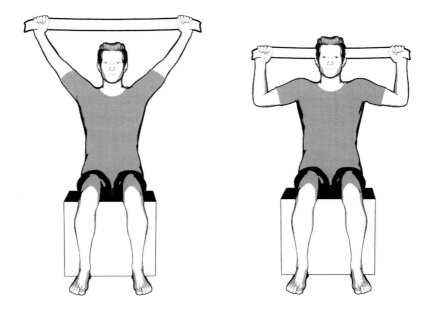

➲ Things to look out for:

▸ Keep the towel taut.
▸ Try not to bend your head forward.
▸ If you can't get the towel behind your head without bending your neck, pull the towel to the top of your head, moving further back as you progress.

Squat and reach: 30 seconds

Start by standing up and using the Moly checklist. Activate your core and make sure your spine is neutral. Bend your elbows and place your hands in front of your chest, elbows behind your hands. Keep your eyes facing forward, fixed on something in front of you.

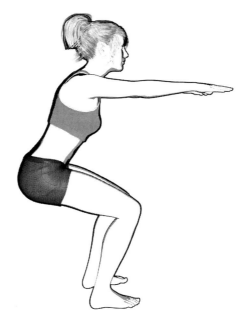

With your feet hip distance apart, toes very slightly facing out, imagine you are sitting down on a chair and push your bottom as far back as you can. At the same time, push your hands forward until your arms are straight. As your bottom goes back, your knees will bend. Make sure your bottom goes no lower than your knees, and your knees no less than a 90-degree angle (thighs parallel to the floor). When you have reached the lowest point of the movement, hold the position for a few seconds, then gently stand back up, bringing your hands back to your chest and bending your elbows.

Repeat this exercise for 30 seconds, breathing in on the way down and out on the way up. To avoid light-headedness, don't do the exercise too quickly.

➲ Things to look out for:

- Keep your eyes facing forward.
- Knees stay behind toes.
- Push your bottom back.
- Maintain a neutral spine.
- You should feel this exercise mainly in your core, thighs and bottom.

The door hinge: 10 on each side

For this you will need a pillow. Lie on your side with your knees bent and your head on the pillow for support. With straight arms, palms together, place your arms out in front of you.

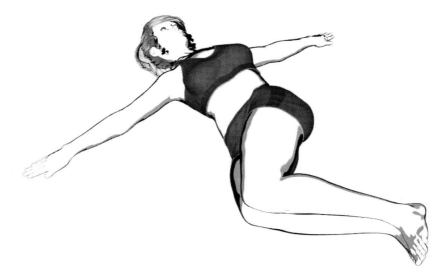

Now, with your legs pressed together and fixed on the floor, move your top arm all the way to the floor behind you. As you do so, let your eyes follow your fingertips. Do the action slowly and in a controlled way. If you rush, you can pull that tight muscle that had been hiding unaware. As soon as the back of your hand hits the floor (whether it is able to depends on your flexibility), take a breath and try to open your chest, stretching your muscles by lowering the active shoulder to the floor. When ready, bring your arm back. Repeat this 10 times on each side.

➲ Things to look out for:

▸ Make sure your eyes follow your hand from start to finish.
▸ Try to keep your knees together, legs on the floor.
▸ Really open your chest when your top hand reaches the floor.
▸ This exercise will show you where is tight and what needs stretching.

The clam: 30 seconds each side

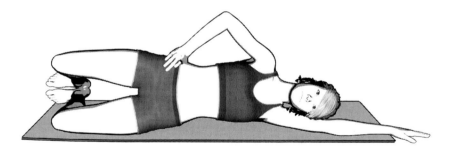

Lie on your side with a pillow or your arms supporting your head. Straighten your legs, with your hips and shoulders in a straight line. Bend your knees so that your lower legs are at a 90-degree angle to your body. Make sure your knees do not travel forward, keeping them in line with your chest.

Making sure you have a neutral spine and your core is activated, tilt your hips slightly forward. If you don't do this, as you begin the exercise, your back will try to take over and you will lose alignment. Keep your feet together and lift your top knee, opening your legs. Then slowly lower the knee back to the start position. Only go as far as you can while keeping your core on and maintaining alignment. Do this exercise for 30 seconds each side.

⮞ Things to look out for:

▸ The golden rule of the clam is that your hips can never be too far forward. This keeps the exercise out of your back and into the gluteus medius.
▸ If the movement is big, you are doing it wrong.
▸ You should feel this in the muscle just behind your hip in the buttock of your top leg.

The bridge: 30 seconds

Lie on your back with your knees bent, feet hip distance apart, arms by your sides. Take in a few deep breaths, relaxing your upper body. Engage your core and, maintaining a neutral spine, take in a breath.

As you exhale, using your core, lift your bottom off the floor, placing your body weight onto your shoulder blades. Tighten your buttocks to lock the position. You will feel a pull on the muscles at the back of your thigh. If you feel anything stronger than a pull, like the muscles beginning to cramp, gently lower yourself down and stretch your hamstrings before trying again. Hold this exercise for 30 seconds.

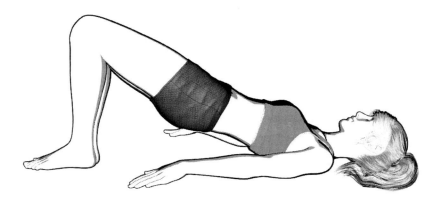

⊃ Things to look out for:

► Keep your core on and buttocks tight.
► If your muscles feel tight, stretch your hamstrings and try again.
► You should feel this exercise in the back of your thighs.

Now let's stretch: Hold each stretch for 20 seconds

Please use the reference at the back of this book and do the following stretches:

► Chest stretch
► Calf stretch
► Quad stretch
► Hug the tree stretch
► Glute stretch
► Gluteus medius stretch
► Hamstring stretch
► Cat stretch

Muscles and joints

For the benefit of those of you who haven't read my first book, *A Better You in Later Life*, an isolation exercise targets one specific muscle group or joint. (It doesn't mean an exercise you do on your own.) The following isolation exercises are designed to build better muscles and joints as part of being An Even Better You.

Static quad raise: Hold for 30 seconds each leg

Lie on your back with your knees bent, feet flat on the floor. Straighten one leg along the floor and place a rolled-up towel under that knee. You do this to make sure you don't overextend your knee, which will pull the muscles behind it. In order to maintain a neutral spine, the leg you are not using should stay bent at a 45-degree angle, with your foot flat on the floor. This helps to prevent you arching your back as you raise your leg. Keep your hands on your chest and make sure your neck is comfortable.

Using the straight leg, point your toes towards your body to activate the calf and lock your leg into position. Make sure your leg is in the correct position by checking the midline (toes, knee and centre of thigh line up) and activate your core. Take in a breath and, as you exhale, raise your leg off the floor a few centimetres and hold it there for 30 seconds. Repeat with the other leg.

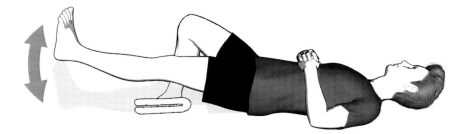

➲ Things to look out for:

▶ Keep your foot dorsiflexed, toes pointing towards you.
▶ Keep your leg aligned by imagining drawing a line straight down the centre of your thigh, knee and foot.
▶ You should feel this exercise in the front of your thigh.

Single leg bridge: Hold for 10 seconds each leg

As before with the bridge, lie on your back with your knees bent, feet hip distance apart, arms by your sides. Take in a few deep breaths, relaxing your upper body. Engage your core and, maintaining a neutral spine, take in a breath. As you exhale, using your core, lift your bottom off the floor, placing your body weight onto your shoulder blades. Tighten your buttocks to lock the position. Then, concentrating on your core and neutral spine, without tilting your hips, straighten one leg by taking the foot off the floor. Keep your thighs and knees together so the only joint that moves is your knee. You now have your bodyweight in just one hamstring, which is difficult, so this may feel really strong. If the leg cramps, stop, stretch and try again. Otherwise hold for 10 seconds and then repeat on the other side.

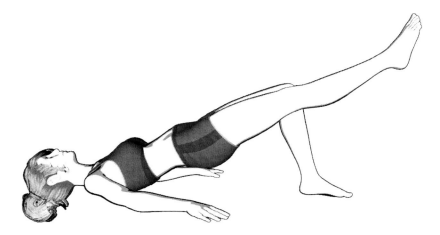

⟳ Things to look out for:

▸ Time to use that core!
▸ Don't let your hips tilt.
▸ Make sure your active leg stays at a 45-degree angle.

Heels off the floor: Repeat 10 times

Lie on your back, knees bent, feet flat on the floor, with your arms by your sides. With a neutral spine engage your core. Try not to strain, but pull in just enough to feel your muscles.

Now, using both legs, keep your heels on the floor and raise your toes. Making sure you keep your core on, now raise your heels slightly off the floor, about the height of a closed fist. When doing this, keep your knees in the same position so the exercise comes from your hip. Lower, then repeat 10 times.

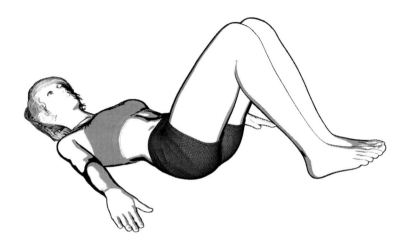

➲ Things to look out for:

▸ Only raise your heels a little off the floor.
▸ You should feel this in the deep muscles between your groin and navel. You should never feel this exercise in your back.

Legs 90 degrees: Hold for 30 seconds

Still lying on your back, place your feet on the floor with bent knees, arms straight by your sides. With an activated core, raise your legs in the air, keeping your knees at 90 degrees and your lower legs parallel to the floor. Push your feet away from your body just enough to feel your core take the load of your legs.

If you feel it in your back it is because your core is not activated and your back has arched. To avoid this, don't push your legs too far away. Hold for 30 seconds.

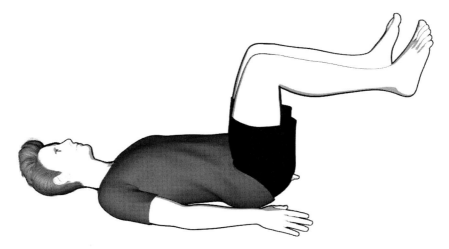

➲ Things to look out for:

► Relax your upper body and activate your core.
► You should feel this exercise in the deep muscles between your groin and navel and maybe in your thighs and hips. You should not feel it in your back.

Clam: 1 minute each side

Lie on your side with a pillow or your arms supporting your head. Straighten your legs, with your hips and shoulders in a straight line. Bend your knees so that your lower legs are at a 90-degree angle to your body. Make sure your knees do not travel forward, keeping them in line with your chest.

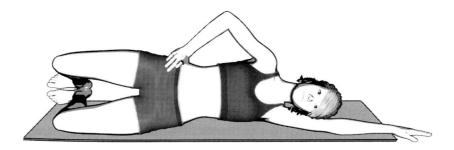

Making sure you have a neutral spine and your core is activated, tilt your hips slightly forward. If you don't do this, as you begin the exercise, your back will try to take over and you will lose alignment.

Keep your feet together and lift your top knee, opening your legs. Then slowly lower the knee back to the start position. Only go as far as you can while keeping your core on and maintaining alignment. Do this exercise for 1 minute each side.

➲ Things to look out for:

▸ The golden rule of the clam is that your hips can never be too far forward. This keeps the exercise out of your back and into the gluteus medius.
▸ If the movement is big, you are doing it wrong.
▸ You should feel this in the muscle just behind your hip in the buttock of your top leg.

The plank: Hold for 30 seconds

Start on the floor on all fours.

Place you forearms on the floor with your elbows directly under your shoulders. Your elbows should be at a 90-degree angle and your hands shoulder width apart.

One at a time, place your feet back, curling your toes under, so that your legs are straight and lifted off the floor. You want to hold a straight line from your heels through to your head, eyes looking at the floor. Activate your core and hold for 30 seconds. If you are struggling to keep a neutral spine and you can feel it in your back, then re-engage your core and raise your bottom a little higher, taking the arch out of your spine.

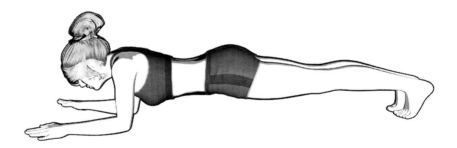

⮊ Things to look out for:

► Keep your elbows directly under your shoulders, hands and elbows the same distance apart.
► You should mainly feel this exercise in your core. If you feel it in your back, activate your core or raise your bottom a little higher.

59

Superman: 30 seconds

Lie on your front with your forehead on the floor. Place your arms out in front of you at full stretch and keep your legs long. Gently and slowly, raise your right arm and left leg, keeping your arms and legs straight. Only a little, just enough to feel them off the floor. Bring them back down and repeat this with the left arm and right leg. Continue alternating sides for 30 seconds.

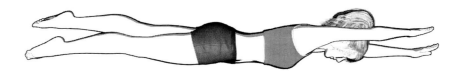

➲ Things to look out for:

► Make sure your arms and legs stay straight.
► Only lift them off the floor a little.
► Keep your head down, forehead on the floor.
► You should feel this in your lower back.

Now let's stretch: Hold each stretch for 20 seconds

► Gluteus medius stretch
► Cat stretch
► Chest stretch
► Quad stretch

Cardiovascular fitness

Time to get your heart rate up!

Interval walking

First of all, I want you to walk for 5 minutes as a warm-up. Walk at a brisk pace, heel to toe, with your core activated. Aim for around 3–5 on the RPE scale. Then find a wall or lamppost for support and stretch each calf for 20 seconds to prepare them for impact. See the stretch references at the end of this book for how to properly do the calf stretch.

Now we are going to implement interval training. This is a really simple way of increasing your fitness and can be done at any level of ability. During the interval training you will alternate between periods of high intensity and low intensity. During the high-intensity phase, you will work out in your aerobic zone, working your heart and lungs, and in the period of low intensity, you will recover. As your fitness improves, you can increase the high-intensity phase and reduce the recovery phase, but for now let's keep it simple. Studies have shown that exercising in this way is just as beneficial as doing longer moderate-intensity workouts, so let's do it!

There are three ways to increase the intensity during a walk: walk faster, walk up an incline or walk up steps.

After the 5-minute warm-up, depending on your ability, body issues or confidence, increase the intensity by walking faster or walking up an incline or some steps, taking your heart rate to the higher end of the target heart rate zone or 5–7 on the RPE scale. Continue doing this for 1 minute, but be sensible. If a minute feels too much, listen to your body and reduce it to 30 seconds. If this is the case, make the minute your goal to build up to. It won't take you long to get there.

After the minute, slow the pace and do recovery walking at low intensity. If you are using steps or an incline, walk slowly back down. The recovery phase can take as long as you like and will depend on your fitness level. The key is that it's a *recovery*. By that I mean that your heart rate should go back down below the target heart rate zone or to 2–3 on the RPE scale. Your goal is to get your heart rate down to recovery in 1–2 minutes.

Repeat the 1-minute high-intensity walk (not the warm-up), then recover again. Do this walk/recover 3–5 times depending on your fitness level.

Now let's stretch: Hold each stretch for 20 seconds

- ▸ Chest stretch
- ▸ Quad stretch
- ▸ Calf stretch
- ▸ Glute stretch
- ▸ Hamstring stretch
- ▸ Cat stretch

Isometric strength training

Just to recap, an isometric exercise targets a muscle without changing its length or using the associated joint.

Straight arm plank: 30 seconds

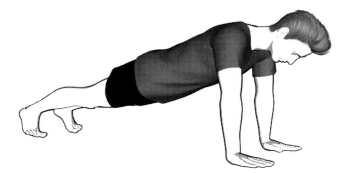

Start by getting down on the floor on all fours. With your fingers facing forward, place your hands directly under your shoulders. Make sure the insides of your elbows are facing each other. Place your legs out behind you, curling under your toes. Tighten your buttocks and activate your core whilst maintaining a neutral spine. Keep your head in line with your back and hold for 30 seconds.

➲ Things to look out for:

- ► Keep your hands directly under your shoulders and your head in line with your bottom.
- ► You should not feel this in your back. If you do, activate your core or raise your bottom a little higher.

Straight arm plank with bent elbows: 10 seconds

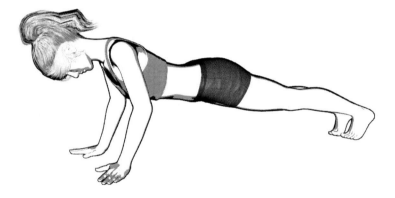

Hold a straight arm plank, take in a breath and lower your body by bending your elbows. Hold your form, keeping your core activated and spine neutral. Your elbows will naturally want to move away from your body, but don't let them. You don't need to bend them a lot, just enough to feel your chest now taking the load of your bodyweight. Try to hold for between 5–10 seconds. Catch your breath and repeat one more time.

➲ Things to look out for:

▸ The more you soften your elbows, the harder it is. The aim is to get to a 90-degree bend at your elbows.
▸ Start by softening your elbows a little, and each time try to go a little further down.

Wall squat: 1 minute

Place your back against a wall, making sure the surface is smooth with no protrusions. Gently walk your feet out to around 60cm (2 feet) from the wall (depending on your height). With your feet just wider than hip distance apart, slide your back down the wall, bending your legs until your knees are at a 90-degree angle (thighs parallel to the floor). Your bottom should not be lower than your knees. Make sure your knees are directly above your ankles, as the closer your feet are to the wall, the more pressure goes into your knees. With your arms straight down by your sides, try to hold this position for 1 minute. When completed, using your thighs, gently and slowly push yourself back up the wall into a standing position.

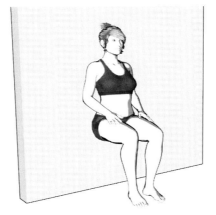

⊃ Things to look out for:

► Keep your hips slightly higher than your knees.
► Make sure your knees are not further forward than your toes.
► Keep your feet at least hip distance apart.
► You should feel this in your thighs.

Squat and reach with hold: Repeat 10 times

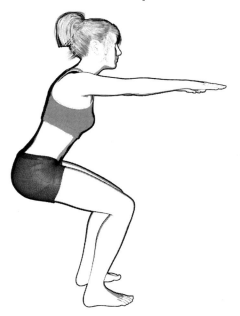

Activate your core and make sure your spine is neutral. Bend your elbows and place your hands in front of your chest, elbows behind your hands. Keep your eyes facing forward, fixed on something in front of you. With your feet hip distance apart, toes very slightly facing out, imagine you are sitting down on a chair and push your bottom as far back as you can.

At the same time, push your hands forward until your arms are straight. As your bottom goes back, your knees will bend. Make sure your bottom goes no lower than your knees, and your knees no less than a 90-degree angle (thighs parallel to the floor). When you have reached the lowest point of the movement, hold the position for 10 seconds, feeling the force in your thighs, core and bottom, not your back. Then gently stand back up, bringing your hands back to your chest and bending your elbows. Repeat this 10 times.

➲ Things to look out for:

- ▶ Keep your eyes facing forward.
- ▶ Knees stay behind toes.
- ▶ Push your bottom back.
- ▶ Maintain a neutral spine.
- ▶ You should feel this exercise mainly in your core, thighs and bottom.

Now let's stretch: Hold each stretch for 20 seconds

- ▶ Chest stretch
- ▶ Quad stretch
- ▶ Calf stretch
- ▶ Glute stretch
- ▶ Hamstring stretch
- ▶ Cat stretch

Increased cardio

Warm-up walk: 5 mins

Walk at a brisk pace, heel to toe, with your core activated. Aim for around 3–5 on the RPE scale.

Interval walk: 1 minute high intensity, 2–3 minutes low intensity (3 times)

As in week 3, work to your target heart rate zones. Walk at a high intensity for 1 minute and then do 2–3 minutes recovery at low intensity. Repeat twice.

Mountain climbers: 10 seconds (twice)

What a great all-rounder this exercise is. Mountain climbers work your core, strength, cardio, balance and coordination; but technique is everything. As great as this is as a one-stop-shop for fitness, if done with poor technique it is equally brilliant at causing harm. So, let's make sure that you get it right.

Start in the straight arm plank position with your hands directly under your shoulders. Alternating your feet, you are going to walk in this position. Bring one foot forward with your knee just off the floor, travelling no further than your hips. Any further than this will lift your back, taking your spine out of neutral. When your knee is at your hips, return your foot to its starting position, maintaining your core and neutral spine. Then repeat the same action with the other leg. Repeat this, alternating your legs, for 10 seconds. Then, have a rest, letting your heart rate settle, and do the exercise again for another 10 seconds.

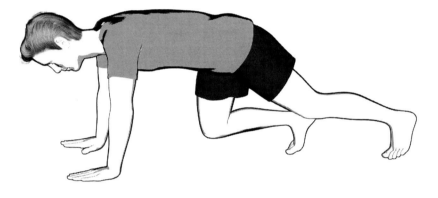

➲ Things to look out for:

This is a tough exercise to do correctly as there are so many things going on at once. Don't forget to breathe. You might find that it hurts your wrists or shoulders. If this is the case, have a look at your technique. Make sure that your hands are not further forward than your shoulders, so your body weight passes directly through your arms. Any further than this will shunt your body weight into your wrists. Also make sure your toes, feet and knees stay in alignment. Avoid letting them do their own thing, flying off to the side.

▸ Keep your core activated and spine neutral.
▸ Make sure your knees do not go past your hips.
▸ Keep your hands under your shoulders.

Plank: 30 seconds

Place you forearms on the floor with your elbows directly under your shoulders. Keep your elbows at a 90-degree angle and your hands shoulder width apart.

One at a time, place your feet back so that your legs are straight and off the floor. Hold a straight line from your heels through to your head, eyes looking at the floor. Activate your core and hold for 30 seconds.

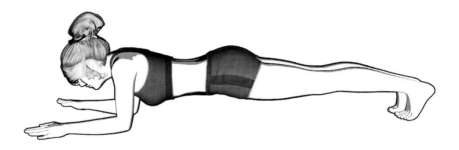

➲ Things to look out for:

▸ Keep your elbows directly under your shoulders, hands and elbows the same distance apart.
▸ You should mainly feel this exercise in your core. If you feel it in your back, activate your core or raise your bottom a little higher.

Now let's stretch: Hold each stretch for 20 seconds

- ▶ Glute stretch
- ▶ Gluteus medius stretch
- ▶ Hamstring stretch
- ▶ Cat stretch
- ▶ Chest stretch
- ▶ Quad stretch
- ▶ Calf stretch

Back to strength

Warm-up walk: 5–10 minutes

Walk at a brisk pace, heel to toe, with your core activated. Aim for around 3–5 on the RPE scale.

Wall squat: 1 minute

Place your back against a wall, making sure the surface is smooth with no protrusions. Gently walk your feet out to around 60cm (2 feet) from the wall (depending on your height). With your feet just wider than hip distance apart, slide your back down the wall, bending your legs until your knees are at a 90-degree angle (thighs parallel to the floor). Your bottom should not be lower than your knees. Make sure your knees are directly above your ankles, as the closer your feet are to the wall, the more pressure goes into your knees. With your arms straight down by your sides, try to hold this position for 1 minute. When completed, using your thighs, gently and slowly push yourself back up the wall into a standing position.

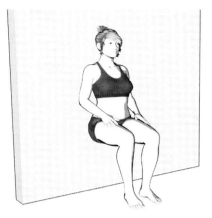

➲ Things to look out for:

▸ Keep your hips slightly higher than your knees.
▸ Make sure your knees are not further forward than your toes.
▸ Keep your feet at least hip distance apart.
▸ You should feel this in your thighs.

Midrow: 1 minute

You will need the tea towel again. Sit in a correct chair (bottom not lower than your knees) with your spine away from the back of the chair so your body weight is supported in your core. Have your feet hip distance apart and your knees bent at a 90-degree angle. Fold the tea towel in half lengthways and then in half again, creating a tea towel bar. Hold the tea towel in front of your stomach with your hands shoulder distance apart, knuckles facing up. Pretend you are about to row in a boat, starting the exercise by pushing your arms straight out at belly button height. Keep your chest open and shoulders relaxed.

Whilst maintaining a neutral spine and activated core, pull the tea towel towards you, bringing it in to your stomach. Keep your elbows tucked in as they travel back, past your chest, squeezing your shoulder blades together. Try not to rock your body. You can prevent this by really working on your core. Your wrists should stay locked in position without rolling, so that only your shoulders and elbows are moving. When you have squeezed your shoulder blades together, straighten your arms back to the forward start position. Repeat for 1 minute.

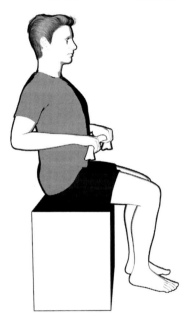

⮑ Things to look out for:

▶ Take your elbows back as far as you can, squeezing your shoulder blades together.
▶ You should feel this mainly in your upper back.

Tea towel behind the neck: 1 minute

Stay seated and hold the tea towel by each end above your head. Keep it taut but don't pull too hard. Now engage your core and make sure your spine is neutral. Keep your eyes facing forward and pull the tea towel down to the base of your neck, keeping it straight without a bend. Then pull it back up again to the starting position. Repeat the exercise for 1 minute.

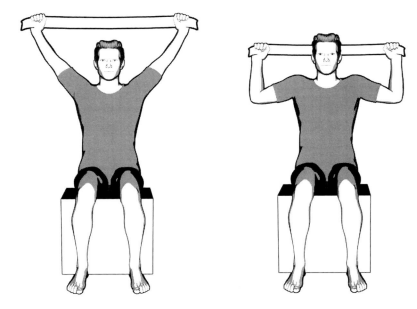

➲ Things to look out for:

- ▸ Keep the towel taut.
- ▸ Try not to bend your head forward.
- ▸ If you can't get the towel behind your head without bending your neck, pull the towel to the top of your head, moving further back as you progress.

Squat and reach: 30 seconds

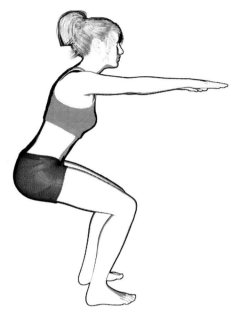

Start by standing up and using the Moly checklist. Activate your core and make sure your spine is neutral. Bend your elbows and place your hands in front of your chest, elbows behind your hands. Keep your eyes facing forward, fixed on something in front of you.

With your feet hip distance apart, toes very slightly facing out, imagine you are sitting down on a chair and push your bottom as far back as you can. At the same time, push your hands forward until your arms are straight. As your bottom goes back, your knees will bend. Make sure your bottom goes no lower than your knees, and your knees no less than a 90-degree angle (thighs parallel to the floor). When you have reached the lowest point of the movement, hold the position for a few seconds, then gently stand back up, bringing your hands back to your chest and bending your elbows. Repeat this exercise for 30 seconds, breathing in on the way down and out on the way up. To avoid light-headedness, don't do the exercise too quickly.

⮥ Things to look out for:

▸ Keep your eyes facing forward.
▸ Knees stay behind toes.
▸ Push your bottom back.
▸ Maintain a neutral spine.
▸ You should feel this exercise mainly in your core, thighs and bottom.

Straight arm plank: 30 seconds

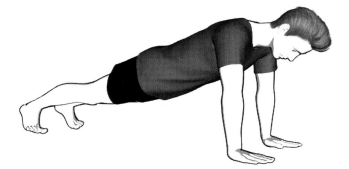

Start by getting down on the floor on all fours. With your fingers facing forward, place your hands directly under your shoulders. Make sure the insides of your elbows are facing each other. Place your legs out behind you, curling your toes under. Tighten your buttocks and activate your core whilst maintaining a neutral spine. Keep your head in line with your back and hold for 30 seconds.

➲ Things to look out for:

- ► Keep your hands directly under your shoulders and head in line with your bottom.
- ► You should not feel this in your back. If you do, activate your core or raise your bottom a little higher.

The bridge: 30 seconds

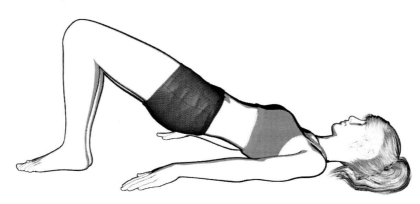

Lie on your back with your knees bent, feet hip distance apart, arms by your sides. Take in a few deep breaths, relaxing your upper body. Engage your core and, maintaining a neutral spine, take in a breath. As you exhale, using your core, lift your bottom off the floor, placing your body weight onto your shoulder blades. Tighten your buttocks to lock the position. You will feel a pull on the muscles at the back of your thigh. If you feel anything stronger than a pull, like the muscles beginning to cramp, gently lower yourself down and stretch your hamstrings before trying again. Hold this exercise for 30 seconds.

➲ Things to look out for:

► Keep your core on and buttocks tight.
► If your muscles feel tight, stretch your hamstrings and try again.
► You should feel this exercise in the back of your thighs.

The clam: 30 seconds each side

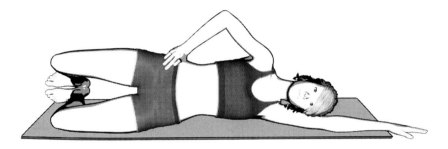

Lie on your side with a pillow or your arms supporting your head. Straighten your legs, with your hips and shoulders in a straight line. Bend your knees so that your lower legs are at a 90-degree angle to your body. Make sure your knees do not travel forwards, keeping them in line with your chest.

Making sure you have a neutral spine and your core is activated, tilt your hips slightly forward. If you don't do this, as you begin the exercise, your back will try to take over and you will lose alignment. Keep your feet together and lift your top knee, opening your legs. Then slowly lower the knee back to the start position. Only go as far as you can while keeping your core on and maintaining alignment. Do this exercise for 30 seconds each side.

➲ Things to look out for:

▸ The golden rule of the clam is that your hips can never be too far forward. This keeps the exercise out of your back and into the gluteus medius.
▸ If the movement is big, you are doing it wrong.
▸ You should feel this in the muscle just behind your hip in the buttock of your top leg.

The door hinge: 10 on each side

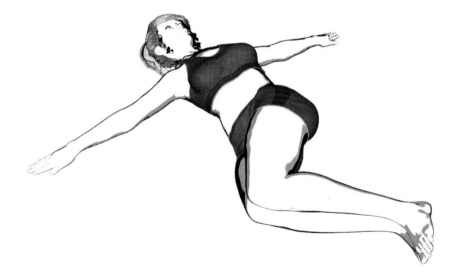

For this you will need a pillow. Lie on your side with your knees bent and your head on the pillow for support. With straight arms, palms together, place your arms out in front of you. Now, with your legs pressed together and fixed on the floor, move your top arm all the way to the floor behind you. As you do so, let your eyes follow your fingertips. Do the action slowly and in a controlled way. If you rush, you can pull that tight muscle that had been hiding unaware. As soon as the back of your hand hits the floor (whether it is able to depends on your flexibility), take a breath and try to open your chest, stretching your muscles by lowering the active shoulder to the floor. When ready, bring your arm back. Repeat this 10 times on each side.

⮑ Things to look out for:

▶ Make sure your eyes follow your hand from start to finish.
▶ Try to keep your knees together, legs on the floor.
▶ Really open your chest when your top hand reaches the floor.
▶ This exercise will show you where is tight and what needs stretching.

Now let's stretch: Hold each stretch for 20 seconds

▶ Glute stretch
▶ Gluteus medius stretch
▶ Hamstring stretch
▶ Cat stretch
▶ Chest stretch
▶ Hug the tree stretch
▶ Quad stretch
▶ Calf stretch

Stretch and core

Pelvic floor: 10 squeezes with a rest in between

It is a common misconception that only women need to do pelvic floor exercises after giving birth. We all need to do them. Pelvic floor exercises strengthen the muscles around your bladder, private bits and bottom, which weaken with age and the menopause.

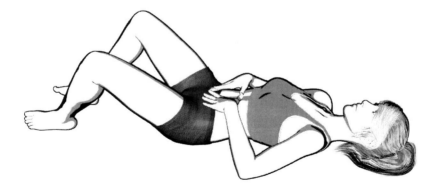

Lie on your back with your knees bent, feet flat on the floor. The best way to understand how to do this is to think about tightening your internals. Imagine you are holding in a wee. Try not to hold your breath. Now isolate your *internal* muscles without tightening your buttocks and stomach. Squeeze those muscles 10 times in a row. When you are used to doing it, try holding each squeeze for a few seconds. It is easy to overdo this exercise so don't do it for too long. Rest for a few seconds between each squeeze!

➲ Things to look out for:

▶ Don't overdo this one.
▶ Try not to let your thighs, bottom and stomach help. Concentrate on isolating your internal muscles.

Diaphragmatic breathing: 2 minutes

Diaphragmatic or belly breathing is great for several reasons. It will:

▶ strengthen your diaphragm
▶ help you relax by lowering stress levels (it can lower cortisol, the stress hormone)
▶ lower your heart rate
▶ help lower blood pressure
▶ help with back pain.

Belly breathing is great for when you have had 'one of those days' and just need a few minutes to yourself to unwind. The technique is simple and straightforward to master, and you can do it sitting or lying down.

Lie on the floor or sit in a correct chair, knees bent and with a neutral spine. Place one hand on your chest and the other on your stomach. Breathe in through your nose, expanding your stomach and letting your belly blow up. Try to limit any movement in your chest and focus it in your stomach. Use your hands to feel the movement in both chest and stomach. Breathe out through your mouth, pulling your belly in. I always breathe in and out to the count of three as that suits me, but you may feel happier with a two or four count. Repeat for a few minutes.

Legs 90 degrees: Hold for 30 seconds

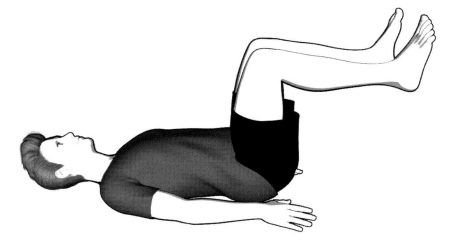

Still lying on your back, place your feet on the floor with bent knees, arms straight by your sides. With an activated core, raise your legs in the air, keeping your knees at 90 degrees and your lower legs parallel to the floor. Push your feet away from your body just enough to feel your core take the load of your legs. If you feel it in your back it is because your core is not activated and your back has arched. To avoid this, don't push your legs too far away. Hold for 30 seconds.

⊃ Things to look out for:

▸ Relax your upper body and activate your core.
▸ You should feel this exercise in the deep muscles between your groin and navel and maybe in your thighs and hips. You should not feel it in your back.

Heels off the floor: Repeat 10 times

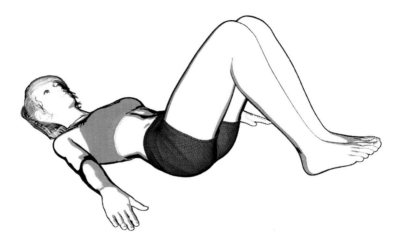

Lie on your back, knees bent, feet flat on the floor, with your arms by your sides. With a neutral spine engage your core. Try not to strain, but pull in just enough to feel your muscles. Now, using both legs, keep your heels on the floor and raise your toes.

Making sure you keep your core on, now raise your heels slightly off the floor, about the height of a closed fist. When doing this, keep your knees in the same position so the exercise comes from your hip. Lower, then repeat 10 times.

⮑ Things to look out for:

► Only raise your heels a little off the floor.
► You should feel this in the deep muscles between your groin and navel. You should never feel this exercise in your back.

Legs 90 degrees with walk: 30 seconds

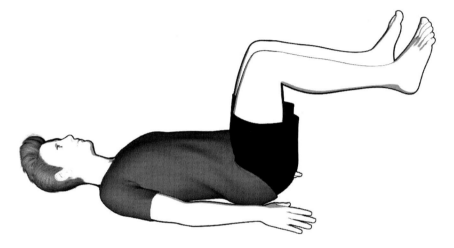

Still lying on your back, place your feet on the floor with bent knees, arms straight by your sides. With an activated core, raise your legs in the air, keeping your knees at 90 degrees and your lower legs parallel to the floor. Push your feet away from your body just enough to feel your core take the load of your legs. Now, with very small movements, start to walk your legs, alternating each leg. Try not to raise or lower your legs, but keep them travelling along the same line. If you feel it in your back it is because your core is not activated and your back has arched. To avoid this, don't walk your legs too far away. Walk for 30 seconds.

Single leg plank: 10 seconds each leg

Place your forearms on the floor with your elbows directly under your shoulders. Your elbows should be at a 90-degree angle and your hands shoulder width apart.

One at a time, place your feet back so that your legs are straight and off the floor. You want to hold a straight line from your heels through to your head, eyes looking at the floor. Activate your core and then, without arching your back, lift one foot off the floor, keeping both legs straight. Keep breathing and hold your form for 10 seconds, then repeat on the other side.

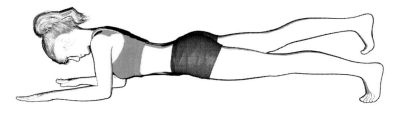

➲ Things to look out for:

▸ Only take your foot off the floor a little.
▸ Try not to tilt your hips, using your core to stabilise the action.

Superman: 30 seconds

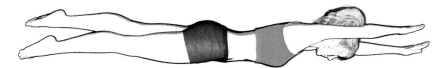

Lie on your front with your forehead on the floor. Place your arms out in front of you at full stretch and keep your legs long. Gently and slowly, raise your right arm and left leg, keeping your arms and legs straight. Only a little, just enough to feel them off the floor. Bring them back down and repeat this with the left arm and right leg. Continue alternating sides for 30 seconds.

➲ Things to look out for:

▶ Make sure your arms and legs stay straight.
▶ Only lift them off the floor a little.
▶ Keep your head down, forehead on the floor.
▶ You should feel this in your lower back.

Now let's stretch: Hold each stretch for 20 seconds

▶ Glute stretch
▶ Gluteus medius stretch
▶ Hamstring stretch
▶ Cat stretch
▶ Chest stretch
▶ Hug the tree stretch
▶ Quad stretch
▶ Calf stretch

Total fitness

Well done for reaching week 8! Now let's bring everything together.

Interval walking: 30 seconds on, 2 mins off (5 times)

First of all, I want you to walk for 5 minutes as a warm-up. Walk at a brisk pace, heel to toe, with your core activated. Aim for around 3–5 on the RPE scale.

After the 5-minute warm-up, find an incline or some steps or walk faster, taking your heart rate to the higher end of the target heart rate zone or 5–7 on the RPE scale. Continue doing this for 30 seconds.

After 30 seconds, slow the pace to recovery walking at low intensity. If you are using steps or an incline, walk slowly back down. Your goal is a recovery period of 1–2 minutes or as long as it takes your heart rate to go back down below the target heart rate zone, or to 2–3 on the RPE scale. Repeat this sequence 5 times.

Mountain climbers: 20 seconds (twice)

Start in the straight arm plank position with your hands directly under your shoulders. Alternating your feet, you are going to walk in this position. Bring one foot forward with your knee just off the floor, travelling no further than your hips. Any further than this will lift your back, taking your spine out of neutral. When your knee is at your hips, return your foot to its starting position, maintaining your core and neutral spine. Then repeat the same action with the other leg.

Repeat this, alternating your legs, for 10 seconds. Then, have a rest, letting your heart rate settle, and do the exercise again for another 10 seconds.

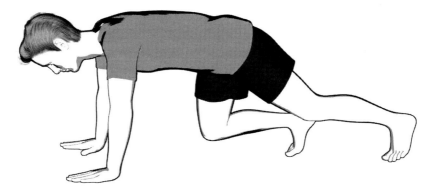

➲ Things to look out for:

▸ Keep your core activated and spine neutral.
▸ Make sure your knees do not go past your hips.
▸ Keep your hands under your shoulders.

Straight arm plank to 90-degree hold: 10 seconds

Start by getting down on the floor on all fours. With your fingers facing forward, place your hands directly under your shoulders. Make sure the insides of your elbows are facing each other. Place your legs out behind you, curling your toes under.

Tighten your buttocks and activate your core whilst maintaining a neutral spine. Keep your head in line with your back, take in a breath and lower your body by bending your arms to 90 degrees at the elbows. Hold your form for 10 seconds, keeping your core activated and spine neutral.

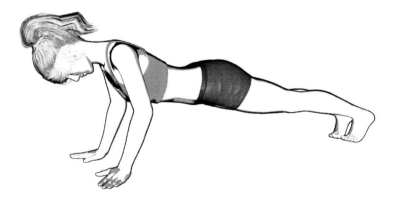

➲ Things to look out for:

▸ Take big deep breaths with this one. Get the oxygen into your body and really use your core muscles.

Single leg bridge: Hold for 10 seconds each leg

Lie on your back with your knees bent, feet hip distance apart, arms by your sides. Take in a few deep breaths, relaxing your upper body. Engage your core and, maintaining a neutral spine, take in a breath.

As you exhale, using your core, lift your bottom off the floor, placing your body weight onto your shoulder blades. Tighten your buttocks to lock the position. Then, concentrating on your core and neutral spine, without tilting your hips, straighten one leg by taking the foot off the floor. Keep your thighs and knees together so the only joint that moves is your knee. Hold for 10 seconds and then repeat on the other side.

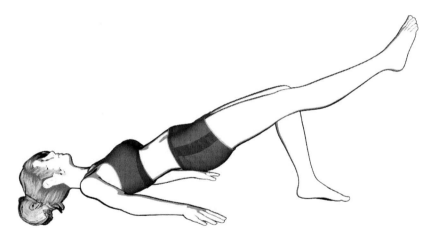

➲ Things to look out for:

► Time to use that core!
► Don't let your hips tilt.
► Make sure your active leg stays at a 45-degree angle.

Legs 90 degrees with walk: 30 seconds

Still lying on your back, place your feet on the floor with bent knees, arms straight by your sides. With an activated core, raise your legs in the air, keeping your knees at 90 degrees and your lower legs parallel to the floor. Push your feet away from your body just enough to feel your core take the load of your legs. Now, with very small movements, start to walk your legs, alternating each leg. Try not to raise or lower your legs, but keep them travelling along the same line. If you feel it in your back it is because your core is not activated and your back has arched. To avoid this, don't walk your legs too far away. Walk for 30 seconds.

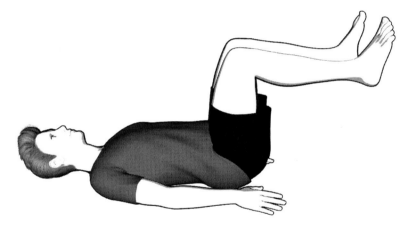

Heels off the floor: Repeat 10 times

Lie on your back, knees bent, feet flat on the floor, with your arms by your sides. With a neutral spine engage your core. Try not to strain, but pull in just enough to feel your muscles. Now, using both legs, keep your heels on the floor and raise your toes.

Making sure you keep your core on, now raise your heels slightly off the floor, about the height of a closed fist. When doing this, keep your knees in the same position so the exercise comes from your hip. Lower, then repeat 10 times.

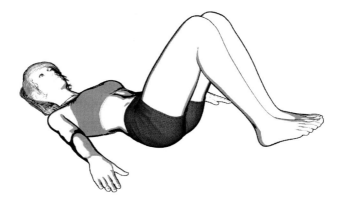

⮞ Things to look out for:

► Only raise your heels a little off the floor.
► You should feel this in the deep muscles between your groin and navel. You should never feel this exercise in your back.

Now let's stretch: Hold each stretch for 20 seconds

► Glute stretch
► Gluteus medius stretch
► Hamstring stretch
► Cat stretch
► Chest stretch
► Hug the tree stretch
► Quad stretch
► Calf stretch

What's next?

I designed the 8-week course to get you back into fitness by exercising every day. Well done for motivating yourself and completing it. The hardest thing about exercise is getting started, getting off your bottom.

Now it has finished, what do you do next? Well, the answer is pick and choose. Take whatever exercises you liked from this book and try to incorporate them into your daily life. You can go back to week 1 and start again or just continue to use one of your favourite daily workouts. It doesn't matter what you choose; what matters is that you exercise daily and get the blood pumping round your body, keeping you healthy.

Remember to listen to your body and that rest is just as important as exercise itself. Sometimes your body just needs some time off, so listen to it. Try not to go more than a few days without exercising or atrophy will kick in and you'll have to start over again.

Be safe and don't forget to keep your core on!

Exercise reference

Moly checklist

Feet hip distance apart

Place your feet the same distance apart as your hips. This will position your feet directly under your hips. Now, make sure that your heels and toes are equal distance apart (feet parallel).

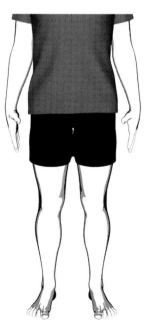

Soft knees

For this you will need to soften, not bend, your knees. You just need to relax your calf muscles slightly, so you feel the tension move out of the back of your legs and into your thighs. If done correctly, you will not feel any pressure in your knees, but just in the front of your thighs.

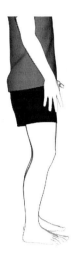

Activate core

Starting from your groin, gently pull your muscles in, up to your navel. Try not to make the action too strong; it should be just enough to feel your muscles activating, not straining. It is easy to overdo this exercise.

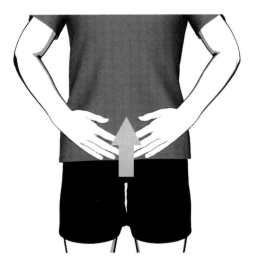

Neutral spine

Here, your lower back should feel comfortable. It should not be too arched, and it should not be too flat. It should be just right. If you are in the correct position then you shouldn't feel your lower back at all.

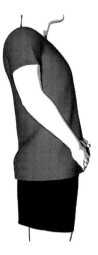

Open chest

Be mindful when opening your chest not to arch your lower back; it is easy to do. When you open your chest, you should feel your rib cage expanding and your shoulders gently travelling back. This will give you the feeling of your chest opening. You should feel the chest muscles opening from your sternum to your shoulders.

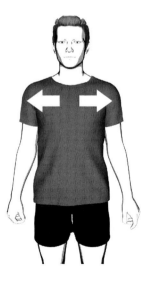

Marching on the spot

When marching on the spot, keep your spine neutral with an activated core.

Keep your elbows at 90 degrees and swing your arms from the shoulder. By swinging your arms, you naturally promote hip swing, which will help raise your legs and (when walking) propel you forward. It also makes your movement more economical, so you will use less energy, enabling you to go further.

Try to get your arms and legs working together. As you raise the right leg, swing the left arm, and vice versa. Again, this will help the movement and make it easier when you are walking.

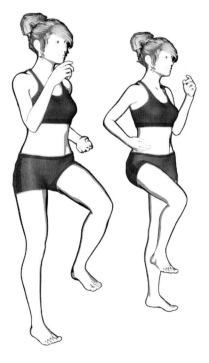

Upper body stretches

Chest stretch

Stand tall with a neutral spine, feet hip distance apart. Open your chest and relax your shoulders. Activate your core. Make a fist behind you in the small of your back and gently try to bring your elbows and shoulder blades together.

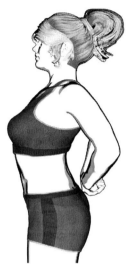

Hold for 20 seconds, taking in big breaths as you do. Breathe in through your nose and out through your mouth. Keep your eyes forward, trying not to bend your neck. You should feel your chest muscles stretching from your sternum towards your shoulders. You may also feel something in your shoulders as they stretch, but look out for pain. If your shoulders are too tight or carrying an injury, the stretch will aggravate it, so be careful and look out for this.

➲ Things to look out for:

► Keep your eyes facing forward and activate your core so that you don't arch your back.
► This is an exercise where you can easily hyperextend your back if your core isn't switched on!

Hug the tree stretch

Stand up with your feet hip distance apart, soften your knees and keep a neutral spine. Imagine that there is a massive tree in front of you with a large trunk and give it a cuddle. Hug it with your fingers clasped together and elbows bent.

Feel your trapezius muscles in your upper back pulling away from each other and pulling outwards away from your spine. Draw that feeling into your shoulders and down your arms. Gently lower your head so you are looking at the floor, as this will stretch the trapezius further. When you are happy that you can feel an effective stretch, hold it for 20 seconds.

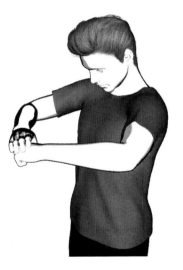

➲ Things to look out for:

► The tree wants to be a big one! Think oak not acer!

Cat stretch

Gently get down onto the floor, onto your hands and knees. With your arms and legs parallel, the same distance apart, arch your spine to the ceiling, pushing your belly up and in. Gently lower your head to stretch your neck. Feel the stretch in the muscles that run from your neck to the base of your spine. Hold this stretch for 20 seconds, and remember to breathe.

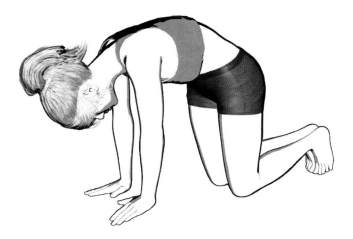

➲ Things to look out for:

► The main area where you should feel this is your back. As you arch up you should feel the muscles stretching on both sides of your spine.
► Keep your head down so the stretch also works in your neck.

Lower body stretches

Calf stretch

Using a wall or something sturdy that can support your bodyweight, place your hands on the wall at shoulder height, keeping your heels under your shoulders so you do not lean in. Take one leg back as far as it will go whilst keeping your heel on the floor. With the front leg, lean your bodyweight forward, keeping your back heel pressed into the floor.

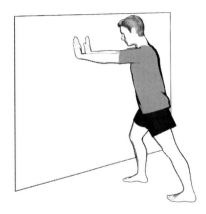

➲ Things to look out for:

► Keep your back heel pressed into the floor

Glute stretch

Lie on your back with your right ankle on your left knee. Keep your shoulders down, relax and breathe. Using both arms, place your hands behind your left leg, just below your bent knee and gently pull your leg towards your chest. Try to keep the angle of your left knee around 90 degrees. You are aiming for your left knee to be above your navel. The stretch should feel strong and obvious in the centre of your right buttock. You should only feel it in the glute. If you can feel it anywhere else, stop. It may be that tight muscles elsewhere are inhibiting the stretch and need to be stretched themselves before you can progress. Don't force it. Hold the stretch for 20 seconds, then repeat with the other leg.

You may not be physically able to take hold of your knee with both hands because of complications elsewhere in your body. If this is the case, place a towel around your leg and pull on the towel to bring your leg towards your chest.

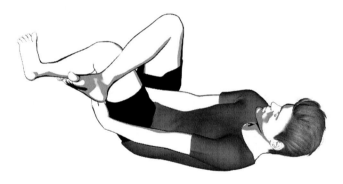

➲ Things to look out for:

- ► Ease into the stretch, don't force it.
- ► Try to keep you head down on the floor.
- ► Keep the leg you are pulling into your body with a 90-degree bend at your knee.

Gluteus medius stretch

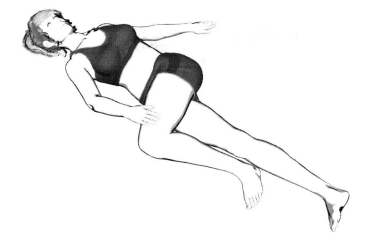

Lie on your back with your right leg flat. Bring your left leg across your right leg and place your left foot so that it is on the outside of your right knee. Make sure the sole of your left foot is not on the floor. You want the inside of your foot and ankle facing the floor. Anchor your body into your left shoulder and place your right hand on your left knee. Gently pull your left knee to the floor. Don't pull too hard or you will turn your pelvis. As soon as you feel a stretch, stop and hold for 20 seconds. Your knee should never touch the floor. It doesn't have to move much to get the stretch. If you try too hard there is a good chance of setting off another muscle somewhere else causing an unwanted spasm. Less is more with this one! Repeat with the other leg.

➲ Things to look out for:

▸ Avoid this exercise if you have had a hip replacement.
▸ Anchor your body with your shoulders.
▸ Your knee should not touch the floor, so don't force it to.

Hamstring stretch

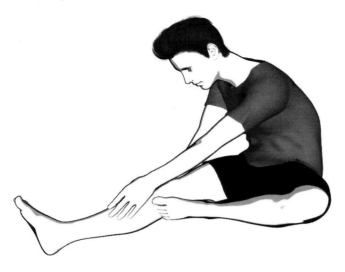

Sit on the floor with your legs out wide. Roll up a towel and place it under your right knee. Place your left foot on the inside of your right knee and, if you can, let your left knee fall down to the floor. Slide both hands down your right leg towards your foot. You should feel this stretch at the back of your thigh, between your knee and bottom. When you feel a strong stretch, hold for 20 seconds. Repeat on the other side.

➲ Things to look out for:

▸ Your active leg (the one you are stretching) should remain soft at the knee, otherwise your calf will take over and you will feel the stretch there instead.
▸ If you can't reach your toes then slide your hands as far down your leg as they will naturally go, hold that position for 20 seconds, then try and slide a little further down towards your foot.

► Alternatively, for a really strong stretch, place a towel around the heel of your active foot and use it to pull yourself towards your foot.

Quad stretch

Support yourself on something appropriate that can fully take your body weight. Standing tall and using the Molyfit checklist, use one hand to bend your leg back at the knee by holding your ankle and taking your foot towards your bottom. The other hand should be holding something suitable for support. Standing tall, when your foot has gone back as far as possible, push your pelvis forward keeping your knees together. Try not to let the bent knee travel forwards. Hold the stretch for 20 seconds, then repeat on the other side.

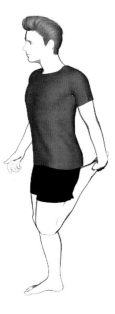

➲ Things to look out for:

► Do not attempt this if you have had a knee replacement.
► If you struggle to grab your ankle, extend your reach by using a towel around your ankle to pull your leg back.
► This stretch should only be felt in your thigh, never in your knee.